CURING BACTERIAL VAGINOSIS NATURALLY

"FINALLY RESOLVE THAT FISHY SMELL!"

Exclusive Bonus Resource for readers of Curing Bacterial Vaginosis Naturally

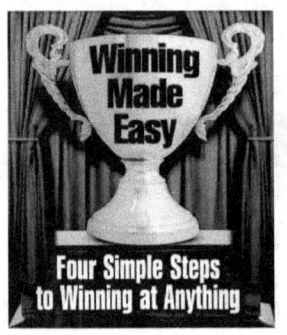

Discover the 4 Steps to Winning Everyday in Every Way in your life!

Learn how you can make money consistently and effortlessly.

Get insider secrets to attracting and keeping your soul mate happy!

Visit http://goo.gl/sQZg9n to claim your above FREE exclusive bonus content.

Contents

What is Bacterial Vaginosis? 3
What Causes Bacterial Vaginosis? 5

    Sperm and Lubricants 5
    Menstruating 5
    Intra Uterine Devices & Scented Tampons 6
    Menopause and Pregnancy 6
    Douching...6
    Antibiotics...6
    Is Bacterial Vaginosis Contagious? 7
    What can cause repeated outbreaks?..7

Signs and Symptoms of Bacterial Vaginosis 8

    Diagnosing Bacterial Vaginosis...8

Risks Associated with Untreated Bacterial Vaginosis..10

    Increased Risk of Infection 10
    Problems with Fertility and Pregnancy..10
    Increased Risk of STDs 10

Treating Bacterial Vaginosis..11
Natural Remedies...12

    Avoid Douching..12
    Liver Detoxification..13
    Reduce Exposure to Toxins 13
    Colon Detoxification...14
    Don't Wash with Soap...14
    Cleansing Bath 15
    Wear the Right Underwear 15
    Breathe While You Sleep...15
    Probiotics and Yogurt 16
    Dietary Changes..16

Simple Detox Recipes 17

    Liver Detox Soup..17
    Liver Cleansing Creamy Soup 18
    Daily Liver Detox Drink...19
    Liver Cleansing Drink...19
    Strawberry Detox Dessert 19
    Colon Detox Juice...20
    Colon Detox Morning Drink..20

Conclusion 21

What is Bacterial Vaginosis?

Bacterial Vaginosis is perhaps one of the most misunderstood feminine problems around. It's often confused with other conditions or infections, which leads it to being commonly misdiagnosed. Not surprisingly, this also means it's frequently treated in the wrong way, which can cause symptoms to persist or to recur in new outbreaks over and over again.

To clear up any confusion in your mind, Bacterial Vaginosis (or BV for short) is simply an unbalanced amount of the natural bacteria we all have within our vaginas. The vagina of every woman on the planet contains a vast number of microorganisms that are required to keep us healthy and to keep everything functioning the way it should.

Unfortunately, there are times when some forms of bacteria tend to become more numerous than they should. This causes an imbalance that creates unpleasant and often embarrassing symptoms that many women dread.

While the symptoms may be unpleasant, BV on its own is not dangerous. It's also not a sexually transmitted disease. It's something that any woman can develop if the right conditions are present within the vagina for bacteria to grow abnormally.

A healthy vagina is usually mildly acidic. Yet in a woman experiencing BV symptoms that acidity is reduced, which stimulates bacterial growth and creates the type of imbalance we're talking about.

Statistics show that approximately 29% of American women have BV. Of the women studied, 60% of women who already had symptoms of a sexually transmitted disease showed BV symptoms. 16% of pregnant women studied also had BV.

Yet it's also estimated that approximately 85% of women with Bacterial Vaginosis experience little to no symptoms at all.

When you consider that BV is nothing more than a simple imbalance within the normal and natural bacteria that is already present within your vagina, it's surprising that medical science insists on treating this condition with pharmaceutical products.

In most cases, patients are prescribed with antibiotics in an effort to stave off the excess bacterial growth. Unfortunately, antibiotics can often cause the same bacteria you're trying to control to grow even faster. This is usually because antibiotics tend to attack 'good' bacteria at the same time as they attack 'bad' bacteria, leading to an even greater imbalance.

This is primarily the reason why so many women who have been diagnosed with BV will experience a recurring outbreak of symptoms very soon after they've completed their course of antibiotic treatment.

Rather than continue to live with embarrassment or shame about Bacterial Vaginosis symptoms, it's very possible to take matters into your own hands. This can be done quite naturally, without the need for medication or antibiotics. It can be done without expensive visits to the doctor's clinic.

What's more, it can be done so that you don't experience frequent outbreaks of symptoms again.

The key is to understand how to get your body working optimally so that it's able to control and regulate the natural bacteria and microorganism growth all on its own.

Are you ready to get started?

What Causes Bacterial Vaginosis?

Despite numerous studies and research conducted around the world, no one is quite certain what the exact cause of Bacterial Vaginosis really is. The current line of thought is that multiple types of certain naturally-occurring bacteria need to be present within the vagina for BV to start developing.

However, studies do show that once a woman has symptoms of BV, the levels of the naturally occurring lactobacilli bacteria that produce hydrogen peroxide are lower than they usually should be. At the same time, studies also show an increase in anaerobic bacteria at very concentrated levels.

Sperm and Lubricants

While researchers can't be certain, there does seem to be a link between having unprotected sex with multiple sexual partners and recurring BV symptoms. However, at the same time it's still very possible for a woman who has never had sexual intercourse before to still develop BV.

Sexually active women having unprotected sex may notice that the fishy smell they're trying to get rid of may get worse after sex. This is because a healthy vagina is supposed to have a pH level of approximately 4. When you have a BV infection, your pH levels rise to around 4.7 or higher.

Sperm has a pH level of 7, which is almost neutral. As mentioned earlier, your vagina is supposed to be slightly acidic in order to remain healthy. Introducing a pH neutral substance into the vagina can make your pH levels even worse, which causes the bad bacteria to grow even more prolifically and make the fishy odor even stronger.

Likewise, some lubricants may be almost pH neutral. If you use lubricants during sexual intercourse, even if you're using a condom, the prolonged presence of a pH neutral substance within the vagina can cause your own pH levels to rise, increasing the risk of more BV symptoms.

Menstruating

Menstrual blood has a neutral pH level of 7.4. When you're menstruating, you are immediately more susceptible to a BV infection simply because the pH levels within the vaginal area are raised. This can cause bad bacteria to grow quickly.

Using tampons may also increase the pH levels within the vagina, as an absorbent tampon will keep the menstrual blood within the vagina for a longer amount of time. It is still safe to use tampons while you're menstruating, but it's very important to change them every 4 to 6 hours to help reduce infection and other complications.

Intra Uterine Devices & Scented Tampons

There may be a connection with the onset of symptoms in women who use an intrauterine device (IUD) for contraceptive purposes. This device can disrupt the natural levels of bacteria within the vagina, causing the unpleasant odor many women with BV worry about.

Likewise, using scented tampons in an effort to reduce any odor during menstruation can actually cause bacterial imbalances that make your symptoms worse.

Menopause and Pregnancy

Some studies have noticed an increase in patients of menopausal age developing BV symptoms. This can be related to the natural hormonal changes occurring in the body during menopause, which can create a bacterial imbalance within the vagina very easily.

Pregnant women also experience fluctuating hormone levels that can trigger the onset of BV symptoms.

Douching

A link may also have been established for BV symptoms in women who regularly use feminine hygiene products to douche. Ironically, many women who douche regularly seem to do so in an effort to reduce or eliminate the fishy odor. They believe a douche will clean the vaginal area and make it less likely to product the offensive smell. Unfortunately, douching may actually be making the symptoms worse.

Many commercially bought douche products contain harmful chemicals, deodorants and artificial fragrances. These can severely affect the naturally occurring bacteria within your vagina. In some people, those chemicals may also cause severe irritation or even infection.

Antibiotics

There is also a link between developing BV symptoms after recently taking antibiotics. This is simply because antibiotics combat a wide range of bacteria within your body, throwing the natural balance out.

Approximately 40% of women using antibiotics to treat BV will experience a recurrence in symptoms between one and six months after they stop taking the medication.

With the last two suspected links, outbreaks may be occurring simply because you're changing your own body's natural ability to regulate normal bacteria on its own. The human body was created with its own regulation systems in place, including your immune system and your natural ability to produce various hormones and secretions that keep everything functioning at its best.

When you interfere with those built-in systems, it's only natural that something will become unbalanced very quickly. Antibiotics may help you to fight off some malicious bacteria, which is why doctors prescribe these when you're fighting an infection. Unfortunately, those same antibiotics can also destroy good bacteria, causing other types of bacteria to grow more rapidly than usual.

Likewise, when you douche regularly you're washing away much of the vagina's natural mucus membranes, which contains many microorganisms you need in order to stay healthy.

At this point, there is no single cause that can bring on BV symptoms. Rather, it seems to be a combination of things working together to cause an imbalance in bacterial flora within the vagina.

Is Bacterial Vaginosis Contagious?

One of the biggest concerns many women have is telling their partner that they have BV. As the condition is so misunderstood, many people instantly jump to the conclusion that it might be a sexually transmitted disease. This can be cause for arguments, mistrust between partners and other personal issues that really shouldn't happen.

The truth is that BV isn't contagious. You can't catch it from a sexual partner and you can't give it to a male sexual partner either. However, BV can be passed between female sexual partners. As mentioned in the previous section, even women who have never had sexual intercourse can still develop BV symptoms.

This can be particularly distressing for younger women and even teenaged girls, who will naturally begin to worry that there's something wrong with them. This isn't true. It's simply one of those conditions that can flourish if the bacteria become unbalanced within your vagina. This can happen to any woman of any age past puberty.

Many urban myths and wife's tales exist about what might cause BV. These include catching it from dirty toilet seats or from swimming in public swimming pools where other 'infected' women might also be present. These aren't true.

What can cause repeated outbreaks?

If you're struggling with BV symptoms coming back regularly, you're not alone. Many women find that if they've had BV once, they're likely to experience a recurrence of the condition at some point.

Many women become embarrassed by their symptoms and may be ashamed to ask a doctor how to treat the symptoms. This usually leads them to doing a little home research on the internet for home-based treatments. Unfortunately, many of those home treatments can end up making the symptoms even worse, especially if they advocate the use of douching.

The key to avoiding repeated outbreaks of Bacterial Vaginosis is to understand how your body works and what's causing the problem in the first place. This makes it much easier to work on positive steps that will help you avoid the condition happening again.

Signs and Symptoms of Bacterial Vaginosis

Even though approximately 85% of women with BV never experience any symptoms, the most distressing and disturbing symptoms other women notice include:

- Abnormal vaginal discharge
- Offensive odor
- Mild itching
- Mild pain or burning sensation when urinating

These symptoms don't seem overly severe on their own, but to the women experiencing them they can be frustrating and embarrassing. In fact, the amounts of vaginal discharge each woman experiences will differ from someone else. The only real indication that your own levels of vaginal discharge may be different will be from your own awareness that something has changed.

In most patients, discharge changes from opaque or clear to a thin, grayish white. This discharge is often accompanied by an unpleasant odor that can be distinctly fishy. It's this odor that usually causes most women to seek treatment in an effort to get rid of it.

In some cases, there may be mild itching around the opening to the vagina. This symptom is what commonly causes people to misdiagnose BV as a yeast infection, or candidiasis. Treatment for a yeast infection won't be effective for treating BV, which is why so many patients complain of frequent recurrences in symptoms.

Some patients also report a mild burning sensation when they urinate. This can often be confused with a mild urinary tract infection or even a yeast infection, which can lead to incorrect treatment for the condition.

Diagnosing Bacterial Vaginosis

It's very common for doctors to misdiagnose BV with a yeast infection. Yet the two are distinctly different conditions that can often present similar symptoms. For most women, the most overt symptom is the distinctly unpleasant fishy odor. This can be uncomfortable and embarrassing for you, but it's not always pleasant for your partner either. This is the main reason most women seek treatment.

In order to accurately treat BV your doctor should conduct a pelvic examination, which should also include an examination of the ovaries and uterus as well. This will help your doctor to rule out any other infections or conditions that may be complicating your symptoms.

Your doctor may take a swab of your vaginal discharge and examine this under a microscope. This type of examination will show a yeast infection very clearly, but it can also show Bacterial Vaginosis, or other types of sexually transmitted infections.

The pH balance of the discharge should also be tested. If the pH levels are higher than 4.5, this can be an indication of BV.

One other examination your doctor may conduct to test for BV is the 'whiff test'. The doctor will combine a small amount of your vaginal discharge with a little potassium hydroxide. The combination of these two things should produce a very strong fishy odor when they're mixed. This gives the doctor a clear indication for a diagnosis of BV.

At this point, your doctor should prescribe you with a course of antibiotics to hopefully clear up the infection.

Risks Associated with Untreated Bacterial Vaginosis

For most women, BV should cause no long term complications at all. Unfortunately, there are some women who may develop some very serious risks, especially if the cause of BV isn't properly treated.

Increased Risk of Infection

If you have untreated BV, you have a much greater risk of developing an infection after vaginal surgical procedures, such as having a hysterectomy or a laparoscopy or an abortion. The bacterial levels within the vagina are already unbalanced and surgical scarring within the area can become easily infected.

Problems with Fertility and Pregnancy

Pregnant women with BV may face an increased risk of premature birth, or of delivering a baby with a low birth weight. Babies born weighing less than 5.5 pounds are considered to be low birth weight. This can put your baby at risk of multiple conditions and problems during important development time.

Women who may be trying to get pregnant may find that BV can create fertility problems. An ongoing untreated BV infection may infect the uterus and even cause fluid to become trapped within the fallopian tubes. This can cause blocked tubes, which makes it impossible for the egg to travel down to the uterus safely. It can also increase the risk of ectopic pregnancy, where the fertilized egg remains trapped within the fallopian tube instead of moving down to the uterus. This condition can be potentially fatal, as it can cause the fallopian tube to rupture.

Increased Risk of STDs

Women with untreated BV have as much more susceptible to contracting other STDs, such as chlamydia, gonorrhea and herpes. What's more, if a woman has unprotected sex with a HIV-infected partner, the chance of contracting HIV infection is greatly increased.

Treating Bacterial Vaginosis

The vast majority of doctors will simply prescribe antibiotics to treat Bacterial Vaginosis. This is their attempt to combat the bad bacteria and stop it from growing so abundantly.

Most patients do report an improvement in symptoms very quickly after taking antibiotics.

Flagyl (or metronidazole) is commonly prescribed as a treatment for BV. This is usually taken in a pill form. This helps to reduce the symptoms almost immediately while you're taking the medication. Metronidazole can also be made available in a gel form called Metrogel, which is applied into the vagina directly. This has also been shown to reduce symptoms very quickly, and has the benefit of having far fewer side effects than taking antibiotics orally.

Your doctor may prescribe a different type of antibiotic, but the same intention is still there. Use of antibiotics to treat an infection is a simple way to get rid of bad bacteria.

However, if you ask anyone who struggles with BV regularly, they'll tell you that the symptoms usually return again after they stop taking the medication. This can happen as soon as one month after stopping the medication, up to 12 months after. Most doctors will simply prescribe another course of antibiotics for these patients and think nothing more of it.

Yet this means antibiotics are not actually curing the problem at all. Rather, they're treating the symptom only temporarily. In some cases, they may actually be making the problem worse.

It's long been known that antibiotics can be effective for fighting off bad bacteria, but it's also well-established that the same antibiotics can also seriously affect the good, or normal, bacteria that you need in order to be healthy.

While taking antibiotics, you may notice that your BV symptoms seem better temporarily. However, it's wise to remember that even the good bacteria you need may have been affected as well as part of your treatment.

Yet when you consider that the vast majority of the causes of BV are based around an imbalance of bacteria within the vagina, taking antibiotics to treat it kind of goes against this logic.

If you're keen to get rid of Bacterial Vaginosis for good, you really need to treat the cause – not the symptom.

Natural Remedies

While your doctor may prescribe antibiotics to treat a BV outbreak, this often only treats the symptoms. It doesn't address the underlying cause and it certainly doesn't address the bacterial imbalance, which means recurring outbreaks are still likely.

Besides, studies have also shown that up to 30% of bacterial vaginosis cases clear up on their own without the help of antibiotic treatments. This means your body is quite capable of correcting the bacterial imbalance within your vagina on its own.

It's also very possible to use some very simple, natural remedies that can actually stop BV outbreaks from recurring and clear up the problem completely. This is usually because you're treating the underlying cause instead of just treating the symptom.

Here are some natural tips and treatments you can try.

Avoid Douching

If you hope to avoid another outbreak of BV, you really need to stop douching immediately. Douching actually interferes with your vagina's natural levels of bacteria, which can decrease the number of good bacteria present and increase the amount of bad bacteria that can cause another outbreak of BV. This has been proven to reduce your risk of conceiving if you douche after intercourse, which is why it may have been used as an unsuccessful method of birth control.

Some commercially bought douche products contain chemicals, deodorants and artificial fragrances that can cause irritation. Yet many people may choose to use plain water, or vinegar diluted in water, or even hydrogen peroxide diluted in water to douche at home. These things may provide short term relief from BV symptoms, but they're not effective over the long term.

Douching frequently with even just water may cause an imbalance in the pH levels within the vagina. This can lead to an increase in yeast infections as well as an increased risk of another outbreak of BV.

Your vagina is naturally slightly acidic. When you douche, you can wash away much of the good bacteria you need that helps keep that natural acidity level. When your pH levels rise by using pH-neutral douches, it makes it much easier for other bacteria to grow more rapidly, causing the imbalance that creates BV symptoms.

Liver Detoxification

Of all the tips you'll find anywhere online, the single most effective way to cure BV symptoms and stop them coming back again is to detox your liver.

Your liver plays a very important role in helping your body to function at optimum levels. One of its primary jobs is to convert any stored body fat into energy. However, it's also designed to remove any toxins out of your system that can cause stress on your immune system. When your immune system is overloaded with toxins, it struggles to fight off any bacterial infections that arise within your body.

For this reason, detoxifying your liver can be the simplest way to get it working optimally again so that your body is more able to restore a healthy balance of bacterial flora within your vagina on its own.

There are some helpful liver detoxification recipes included in a separate section of this book to help you with this step.

Reduce Exposure to Toxins

One of the most predominant reasons your liver struggles so hard to eliminate toxins from your system and keep your immune system healthy is that we're constantly bombarded by chemical toxins in our regular lives.

If you've gone to the effort of detoxifying your liver to get it working at its best, it's also equally as important to take the next step of removing any unnecessary toxins from your daily life.

Cutting out simple things like smoking cigarettes or drinking alcohol can make a big difference to the level of toxins within your body, but there are other household toxins that can adversely affect your liver as well.

These include:

- Mold
- Household cleaning chemicals
- Dust mites
- Cosmetics
- Hair dye
- Food coloring
- Perfumes and chemical-based fragrances
- Air pollution
- Car exhaust fumes
- Pesticides
- Chemical-based fertilizers
- Weed sprays, or herbicides

If you're serious about never having to deal with fishy vaginal odor again in future, you owe it to your body to find ways to reduce the amount of toxins in your immediate environment. This will ensure that your liver is working well and that your immune system becomes stronger. These things combined will make you less prone to recurrent BV infections in future.

Colon Detoxification

The process of detoxifying your body shouldn't just stop at your liver. You also need to consider detoxing your colon as well. After all, you colon is one of the most fertile breeding grounds for bacteria within your body.

Your colon is your body's waste outlet, so it really is important that toxins can be eliminated properly and effectively without any risk of excess bacteria making your system struggle harder than it needs to.

Many of the colon detox diets circulating online advocate fasting or just drinking juice and water to rid your intestines and colon of any toxins. Unfortunately, these types of diets aren't always considered safe or healthy over the long term.

Instead, consider drinking more water throughout every day. Water will naturally get your digestive system and waste elimination system working more effectively. On top of this, find ways to include foods that are high in natural dietary fiber to your diet. This includes green leafy vegetables, fruits, beans, legumes, cereals, whole grains and nuts.

The result of removing many of the toxins that can live within your intestines, bowels and colon can be increased energy levels, and a reduction in bloating and constipation. You should also notice that it's much easier for your body to fight off any future BV infections.

You'll find some easy colon detoxification recipes in a later section of this book.

Don't Wash with Soap

Your vagina was created to be self-cleaning. This means you don't need to use soap or any other feminine hygiene products to wash it. Even if you think you're washing away the fishy smell that comes from a BV infection, you could actually be making the problem worse. You may also be increasing your risk of other infections.

Instead, use water to wash around the labia while you're in the shower or bath.

Cleansing Bath

Run a bath and put 1 ½ cups of apple cider vinegar into the water. Then sit back in the tub and relax for half an hour. Apple cider vinegar is a very mild astringent that can help to regulate pH levels and reduce the over-abundance of bad bacteria that could be causing the offensive odor.

This is also an ideal remedy for recurring yeast infections and urinary tract infections, as this will also help to stop the itching and pain very quickly.

If you have dry skin or eczema, soaking in a bath with apple cider vinegar will also help to relieve these symptoms.

It's important not to use undiluted apple cider vinegar directly on the vaginal area. This will burn and sting and can cause other problems. Simply use 1 ½ cups of apple cider vinegar in a bath tub of water to dilute it. This will be strong enough to help restore the healthy pH levels within your vagina, which will reduce your BV symptoms very quickly and prevent any future outbreaks.

Wear the Right Underwear

Most people believe that wearing cotton underwear is best, simply because cotton 'breathes'. While this might be true, cotton can pose a problem when it gets wet. It takes much longer to dry, which can increase the amount of bacteria in the vaginal area and post a risk of developing fungal infections. If you already have BV symptoms, you may have more discharge than usual, which can cause your underwear to remain wet for longer.

Some modern synthetic underwear doesn't tend to allow as much airflow around the vagina, but it does dry very quickly. This means you actually have a slightly lower risk of infection developing due to wetness. Unfortunately, with polyester fabrics there is still the humidity factor to consider, as there is still a lack of airflow to the area and there's a tendency for polyester to lock in moisture, which can increase yeast infections and BV outbreaks.

If you're in doubt, opt for cotton underwear whenever possible. If you have problems with wetness, consider using a panty liner throughout the month to draw moisture away from your vaginal area and change this regularly to reduce risk of other infections.

Breathe While You Sleep

Whenever possible, don't wear underwear to bed. This allows more airflow around your vagina throughout the night. When you wear underwear all night you reduce the amount of oxygen that can reach the area. This increases humidity levels in the vagina region and can cause an increase in the amount of bacterial flora that develops, can cause fungal infections, and can increase irritation.

It's best to go without when you're heading off to sleep!

Probiotics and Yogurt

If you already have a bacterial imbalance within the vagina, chances are you're likely to have other imbalances within your body as well. For this reason, it can be very beneficial for some women to add multi-strain probiotics to their regular diet. These can be taken in the form of capsules available at your local health food store.

Yogurt does contain lactobacillus, but this isn't the right strain you need in order to treat BV. It's still a good idea to include some natural yogurt in your diet or in some cooking recipes anyway. Not only will this help your body to start regulating bacteria within your gut and your intestines, but it can also help your body get your vaginal pH balance back to normal on its own as well. Yogurt does still contain active cultures that help to boost your immune system and digestive system healthy, so you're still doing your body a favor.

Dietary Changes

Many American women simply don't get enough of the right types of nutrients, vitamins and minerals they need in a balanced diet in order to stay healthy. This simple fact alone can be one reason why your body isn't able to naturally fend of BV infections.

Add more fresh vegetables and fruit to your diet and drink more water each day. Work on ways to reduce the amount of processed or pre-packaged foods you eat. Reduce the amount of sugar in your diet, as sugar can increase your body's pH balance overall.

Eating fresh vegetables can be a great way to get more of the right nutrients your body needs to function properly. Increasing your water intake can seriously help your body to flush out toxins more effectively. Look up simple recipes you can make that include healthier food choices and experiment with foods you enjoy.

These simple things alone won't cure BV, but you'll be creating a healthier body and a healthier immune system that will be more capable of fighting off future infections more easily.

Simple Detox Recipes

The whole idea of detoxifying your body is to help restore a healthier, more efficient balance for your vital organs. The result of this simple step can be astonishing.

You should find that you have more energy after a liver or colon detox. You'll wake up feeling refreshed. Your immune system will be stronger and more able to fight off infections. Your brain function may improve, giving you a clearer mind and improved memory recall.

Most importantly, you should notice that it's much easier to avoid recurring BV symptoms naturally.

Many people feel more comfortable about purchasing specific detox programs, pills or shakes from a pharmacy for this step. Others feel that they need to follow a strict, restricted diet for several days to get any effects at all.

The truth is, it's possible to add detox recipes into your regular diet plan. If you're actively working on ways to include healthier food options and more nutrient-rich foods into your diet to help boost your immune system, you may only need to add some cleansing and detoxifying recipes into your weekly plan to help your liver flush out any excess toxins.

The ingredients used in these recipes actively help your liver to produce beneficial enzymes that help it to flush out any toxins more easily.

Here are some simple detox recipes you can use to keep your body as healthy as possible:

Liver Detox Soup

Ingredients:
- 4 potatoes
- 4 carrots
- 2 sticks celery
- 3 whole beets
- 2 onions
- ½ bunch spinach or silverbeet
- 1 cup green beans
- 10 cloves garlic
- Olive oil
- 8 cups water

Method:

Chop all of the vegetables into bite sized chunks, shred the spinach finely and crush the garlic. In a medium-large saucepan, add the olive oil, garlic and onions and sauté lightly for a few minutes over a medium heat.

When onions have softened, add the water and all the vegetables. Bring the soup to the boil. When it begins to boil, reduce the heat and allow the soup to simmer for 40-50 minutes or until all vegetables are soft.

Serve and eat immediately. Any leftover portions can be frozen for up to 3 months in an air-tight container for future use.

Liver Cleansing Creamy Soup

Ingredients:
- 1 onion
- 3 cloves garlic, crushed
- 2 cups cauliflower
- 2 cups broccoli
- ½ bunch spinach
- 6 cups water
- 5 chicken stock cubes
- ½ teaspoon dried paprika
- ½ teaspoon dried basil
- Olive oil

Method:

Chop all vegetables roughly before you begin. In a medium-large saucepan, add olive oil, onions and garlic and sauté lightly over a medium heat. When onions have softened, add the water, stock cubes and other vegetables.

Bring the soup to the boil. When it's boiling, reduce the heat to low and allow the soup to simmer for 20 minutes, or until all the vegetables are soft.

Remove the soup from the heat and use a stick blender to blend everything until it's smooth and creamy. Serve immediately.

Any remaining portions of this soup can be frozen in an air tight container for up to 2 months for future use.

Daily Liver Detox Drink

Ingredients:
- 2 tablespoons olive oil
- 2 cups freshly squeezed orange juice
- 1/3 cup freshly squeezed lemon juice
- 2 cloves garlic, crushed
- 1/2" fresh ginger
- Pinch of cayenne pepper

Method

Place all the ingredients into a blender and blend until everything is well combined. Drink this mixture every day to keep your liver healthy.

Liver Cleansing Drink

Ingredients:
- 2 apples, chopped and cores removed
- 5 carrots
- Juice from 1 lemon
- 1 ounce fresh beetroot
- Handful of dandelion greens

Method:
Place all the ingredients into a blender and blend until everything is well combined. Drink this mixture at least once a week to help cleanse your liver.

Strawberry Detox Dessert

Ingredients:
- ½ pound strawberries, chopped
- 1 cup silken tofu, chopped
- Grated orange peel from ½ an orange
- 1 teaspoon honey

Method:
Drain the tofu, chop and grate the other ingredients, and place everything into a blender. Blend the mixture until everything is well combined. Pour into dessert bowls and refrigerate for 30 minutes before serving.

Colon Detox Juice

Ingredients:
- 2 apples, cores removed
- 2 spinach leaves
- 2 sticks celery
- 2 carrots
- 1 cup freshly squeezed orange juice

Method:
Add all the ingredients into a blender and blend until smooth. Drink every morning to help flush toxins out of your bowel and colon.

Colon Detox Morning Drink

Ingredients:
- 10 ounces water
- 2 tablespoons freshly squeezed lemon juice
- 2 tablespoons grade B maple syrup
- Pinch of cayenne pepper

Method:
Mix all the ingredients together in a tall glass. Drink this first thing in the morning to kick start your metabolism and to flush out your digestive tract and your colon very effectively.

Conclusion

If you've struggled with Bacterial Vaginosis symptoms and haven't had any luck in getting rid of your symptoms, hopefully this book can help you. Once you find a way to balance the bacterial flora levels within your vagina, you should find it's much easier to avoid any recurring outbreaks of symptoms.

The key is always to remember that you're aiming at maintaining a healthy balance of microorganisms and bacteria at all times. Take a close look at your current food and diet choices and see where you might make small changes that help you to get more nutrient-rich ingredients into your meals.

Look for ways to increase your water intake and actively avoid anything that puts you at risk of any future BV outbreaks.

Before long, those embarrassing, annoying, frustrating BV symptoms you struggled with for so long will be a distant memory.

Here's to your good health!